Inventors and Creators

Jonas
Salk

Other titles in the Inventors and Creators series include:

Inventors and Creators

Jonas
Salk

Deanne Durrett

KIDHAVEN PRESS

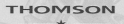

THOMSON
™
GALE

Detroit • New York • San Diego • San Francisco
Boston • New Haven, Conn. • Waterville, Maine
London • Munich

On cover: Jonas Salk in his lab.

Library of Congress Cataloging-in-Publication Data

Durrett, Deanne, 1940–
  Jonas Salk / by Deanne Durrett.
    p. cm. — (Inventors and creators)
  Includes bibliographical references and index.
Summary: Profiles the man who made his mark as developer of a
polio vaccine, struggled to deal with the resultant fame, and emerged
as a philosopher/scientist, writing and speaking about our
responsibility for the future.
  ISBN 0-7377-1277-5
  1. Salk, Jonas, 1914–1995 Juvenile literature. 2. Virologists—
United States—Biography—Juvenile literature. 3. Poliomyelitis
vaccine—Juvenile literature. [1. Salk, Jonas, 1914–1995   2. Scientists.
3. Poliomyelitis vaccine.] I. Title. II. Series.
  QR31.S25 D87 2002
  610'.92—dc21

2001006213

Contents

Research Genius

American scientist Jonas Salk developed the first successful polio **vaccine**. Although other scientists found pieces to the puzzle, Jonas Salk slipped each piece in place and found the solution. America credits him with conquering polio and remembers him as the man who saved children from this dreaded disease.

Before the Salk vaccine became available in 1955, summer brought polio season. Epidemics spread across America and other parts of the modernized world. The disease struck mostly children. Many recovered without any lasting effects. Far too many, however, died. Some were severely paralyzed and could not breathe outside an iron lung (a machine that forced air in and out of the lungs). And, the disease left thousands of children with deformed limbs and twisted bodies. Many of these would never leave their beds except in wheelchairs or assisted by leg braces and crutches.

Jonas Salk freed children from this threat and their parents from the fear of polio. People who remember

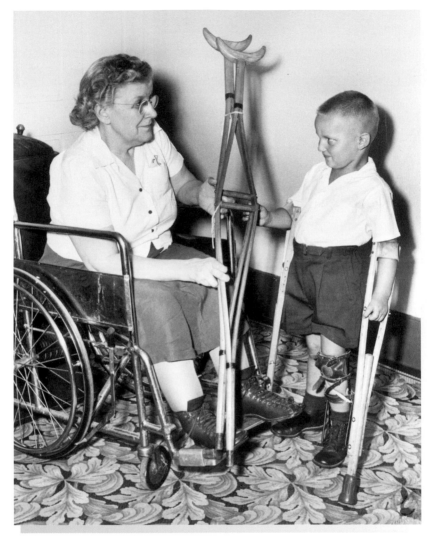

A boy with polio stands next to the first known victim of polio in the United States.

polio (and some of those who don't) consider the Salk vaccine the most important science and technology advancement of the 1950s.

Chapter One

A Boy with Potential

Jonas Edward Salk was born on October 28, 1914, in New York City. He was the first of three sons born to Russian-Jewish immigrants Daniel and Dora Salk. Daniel Salk worked in New York's garment district, where much of America's clothing was made.

Dora and Daniel Salk had little formal education, but they wanted their sons to succeed and considered education a must. With this in mind, Dora became the driving force in the Salk boys' lives.

Recognizing that Jonas was bright and responsible, Dora Salk expected perfection from him and held him to high standards. She demanded more and more of him; every time he reached one goal, she set another. As a result, Jonas believed that he could always do better. He learned to be observant, independent, and thorough in his studies. Even as a child, when Jonas stated something as fact, the adults around him knew he was right. Displaying his independence and confidence, he once said, "Someday I shall grow up and do something in my own way, without anyone telling me how."[1]

Salk as a Student

When he was twelve years old, about the time most students finish sixth grade, Jonas skipped ahead two grades and enrolled at Townsend Harris High School. This New York City school for gifted boys required its students to finish high school in three years instead of the usual four. Jonas did just that.

In 1929, at the age of fifteen, he enrolled in City College of New York. Upon graduation, he planned to go to law school. Until his college years, Jonas had shown little interest in science. His only experience had been a

Even as a boy Jonas Salk was observant and independent.

physics class at Townsend Harris. College-level science courses, including chemistry and biology, however, opened his eyes to a new and exciting world. He was fascinated by the nature of plants, animals, and microscopic creatures. With his logical mind and sense of order he felt well suited to chemistry. By the time he graduated from City College in 1934, he had dropped his plans for law school and decided on a medical career. He enrolled at the New York University School of Medicine that same year. The Salks borrowed money to pay Jonas's first-year tuition. After that he earned scholarships and took part-time jobs for extra money.

Laboratory Experience

During his second year of medical school, Jonas received a fellowship to work in a **laboratory** full time. He studied bacteria and viruses. By this time, other scientists had developed vaccines to prevent typhoid and diphtheria, life-threatening diseases caused by bacteria.

They made these vaccines from killed bacteria, which cannot cause the disease. Still, the patient's body recognizes the injected killed bacteria as a threat. The immune system custom designs a protein, called an **antibody**, and releases it in

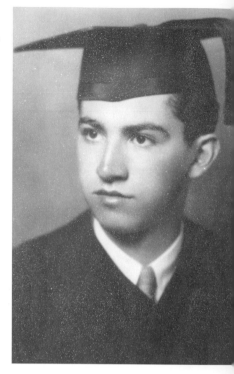

At age nineteen, Salk entered medical school after his graduation from City College in 1934.

the bloodstream to destroy the bacteria. These proteins remain in the bloodstream ready to defend the body from that bacteria. The person is said to be **immune** to that disease. Preventing disease caused by a virus, however, was thought by most to require a **live virus vaccine**. The way to create a successful live virus vaccine against polio, however, remained a mystery.

Excited by the challenges found in the laboratory, Salk soon decided to become a research scientist. When Salk told his classmates he planned to go into research, they could not understand why he would give up the good income from a medical practice for the small salary that a research scientist would earn. Salk, however, would not change his mind. He loved research and would find his life's work in the laboratory. A few years later, he was asked why he had dedicated his life to research. He replied with a question, "Why did Mozart compose music?"[3]

Enlightenment

The next year, 1936, Jonas Salk went back to the classroom. In one class, his professor said that diseases caused by bacteria could be prevented with a vaccine created from the killed bacteria. In the next class, however, another professor assured the young medical students that the only way to prevent diseases caused by a virus was for the patient to be infected by a living virus. These two professors made an impact on Jonas Salk that he would not forget. He later said, "I remember exactly where I was sitting, exactly how I felt at the time—as if a light went on. I said, 'Both statements can't be true.'" In later years, he proved one was not.

The Influence of World Events

During Jonas Salk's youth, everyone, including the Salk family, lived in fear of disease. When Jonas was two years old, an outbreak of polio swept across the United States. Twenty-seven thousand reported cases made the outbreak of 1916 the nation's first polio epidemic. More than nine thousand cases were reported in New York City alone. Because most polio victims

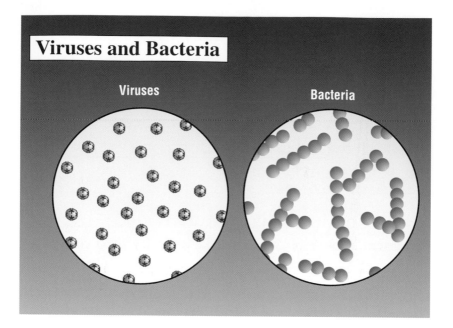

Viruses and Bacteria

Viruses

Bacteria

were children, the disease was also known as **infantile paralysis**. Many victims who survived never walked again. Others wore leg braces and used crutches the rest of their lives. No one knew what caused polio or how the illness was carried and spread. They soon learned that polio epidemics came every summer. People were urged to avoid crowds and health officials closed public swimming pools, playgrounds, and movie theaters. Parents kept their homes very clean. Doors and windows were kept tightly closed. Still, the disease spread.

In 1918, two years after the first U.S. polio epidemic, another deadly disease spread around the world. The influenza pandemic (worldwide epidemic) struck just as World War I ended. The United States lost thousands of troops overseas to the illness and more than five hundred thousand Americans died at

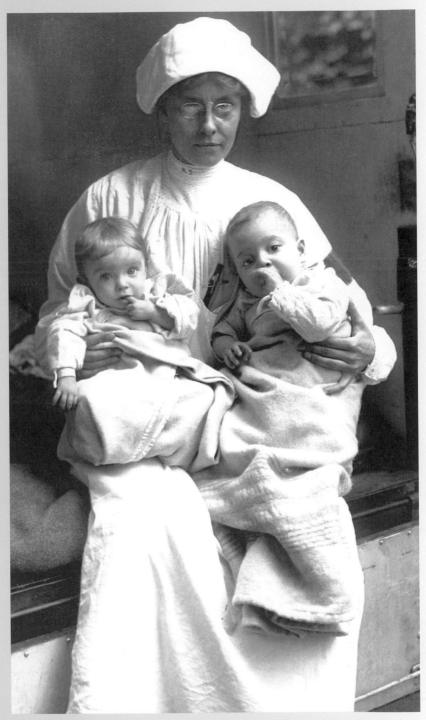

A nurse cares for two young victims of polio in 1916.

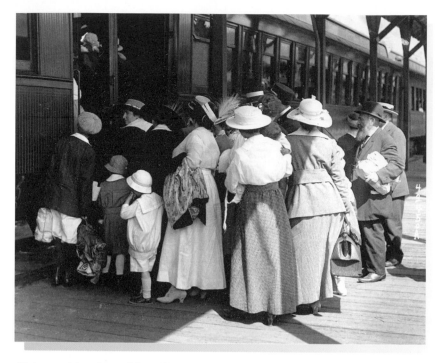

Gripped by fear, New Yorkers flee polio in 1916.

home. Like polio season, influenza struck annually, but its season was winter.

Through much of the first half of his life, Jonas witnessed the fear that gripped America, summer and winter, as these epidemics arrived each year. During this time, research scientists were well on their way to controlling diseases caused by bacteria. Salk would one day be instrumental in the long battle to conquer diseases caused by viruses.

Chapter Two

Man of Opportunity

Throughout his early career Jonas Salk seemed to be in the right place at the right time to gain the experience, knowledge, and financial support he would need to develop the first polio vaccine. He did not, however, desire riches and fame. He was intrigued by science and wanted to discover its secrets to prevent disease and save lives.

Medical School Research

During his senior year at New York University medical school, students were allowed a two-month work-study program in the field of their choice. Salk chose laboratory research and was assigned to work with Dr. Thomas Francis Jr. A top-ranked microbiologist, Francis believed, as Salk suspected, that an effective vaccine could be produced from a killed virus. At the time, Francis was working with another scientist, Dr. George Levin, at the nearby Rockefeller Institute. They experimented with the influenza (flu) virus by exposing it to ultraviolet (UV) radiation. They wanted to know if the influenza virus killed in this way would trigger the body's production of antibodies well enough to provide protection against the disease. Salk had the opportunity to work with both these scientists and took part in every aspect of the experiment. He later said, "It was excellent preparation for later studies and later ideas."[4]

Graduation, Marriage, and Research

In his spare time between the institute and university labs, Jonas Salk dropped by the New York School of Social Work to see Donna Lindsay. He was there so often that some people

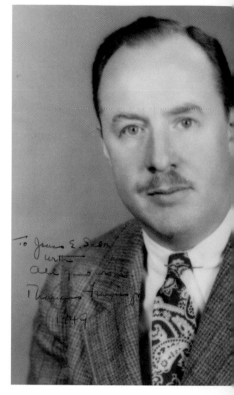

Dr. Thomas Francis Jr. (pictured) guided Salk's early work.

thought he was a student. He was not studying, however, he was falling in love. Salk graduated from New York University School of Medicine on June 8, 1939, and married Donna the next day.

The young couple made their first home in an apartment in New York. Jonas and Donna would have three sons: Peter (born in 1944), Darrell (1947), and Jonathan (1950). This marriage, however, would end in divorce in 1968. Jonas Salk would marry again in 1970, this time to Francoise Gilot, who shared his interest in art.

Soon after graduating from medical school and his marriage to Donna, Salk received a grant ($100 a month) from the Rockefeller Foundation. As a result, he continued his work on ultraviolet irradiation with Francis and Levin until March 1940, when he entered the next phase of his training.

A Salk family photo, summer 1957. Jonas stands at far left.

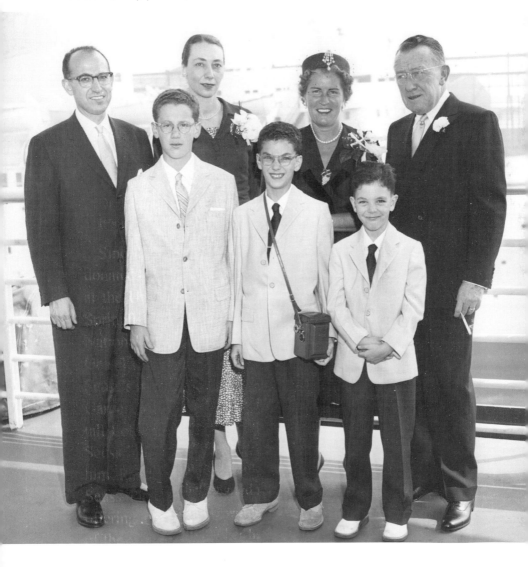

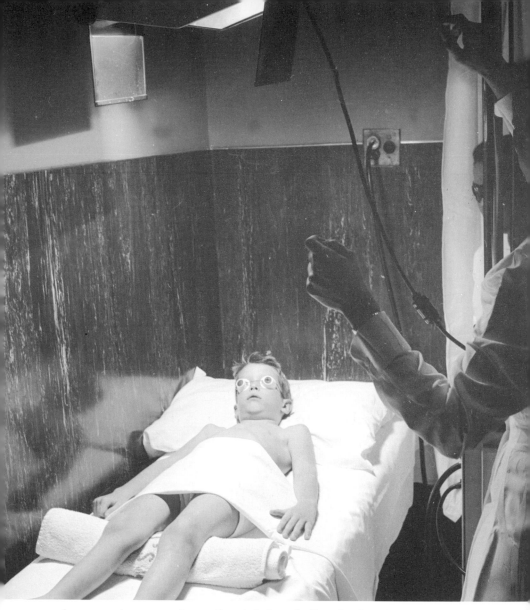

A young boy receives ultraviolet radiation for treating polio in the 1950s.

Mt. Sinai Intern

Salk applied for an internship at Mt. Sinai Hospital in New York City. This top-rated hospital chose twelve of the best medical school graduates to enter their intern program each year. Jonas Salk was one of the twelve selected in 1940.

During his two years at Mt. Sinai, Salk was described as the best intern in the hospital. He was reliable and a perfectionist, with a talent for accurate diagnosis (determining the patient's illness). He was warm, charming, and sympathetic toward his patients. In addition, he displayed surgical skill that brought him invitations to join established medical practices and earned the respect of other interns. All these qualities would have made him an excellent physician in private practice and elevated him among his peers. Still, private practice did not interest Salk; he remained committed to a career in research.

Job Search

By the time Salk completed his internship in 1942, he had decided to do research in the field of viral diseases such as influenza and polio. Although he wanted to stay in New York, Salk's job search led him back to his mentor Thomas Francis.

Francis had moved to the University of Michigan in 1941, where he continued his work with the influenza virus. Besides being employed by the university, he received funding from the National Foundation for Infantile Paralysis (NFIP) to study polio epidemics.

There was no university position available to Salk at this time. Francis, however, recommended him for a fellowship grant to work with him in developing an influenza vaccine. Approved for an annual grant of $2,100, Salk began work with Francis at the University of Michigan on April 12, 1942.

A Matter of National Security

Four months earlier the United States had entered World War II, and now the military considered Francis's work on the influenza vaccine a matter of national security. (More U.S. troops died in the 1918 influenza epidemic than were killed in battle during World War I.) Fearing that testing a live virus vaccine might cause an outbreak of flu among the troops, military planners favored Francis and his research on a **killed virus vaccine**.

A Recognized Expert

During the five years Salk worked with Francis, he participated in most aspects of the research, including developing and testing the vaccine and studying the results. In their work, Salk and Francis learned that influenza is caused by several strains (varieties) of the influenza virus. This was the key to creating a successful influenza vaccine. Salk later explained that to make a successful influenza vaccine, "You must cram your vaccine with every strain you can lay hands on."[5] As a result of their dedicated effort, Salk and Francis developed the first successful influenza vaccine.

Salk's work with Francis involved only the influenza vaccine, not polio research. However, NFIP was aware of his work. And, the young scientists impressed them.

While involved in the influenza research at the University of Michigan, Salk acquired knowledge, technical know-how, and deeper understanding of the way the immune system fights disease. In addition,

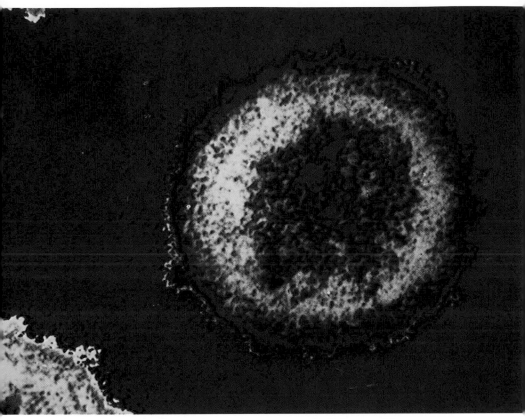

A virus as seen through a microscope. Salk hoped to conquer viral diseases.

Salk had a talent for analyzing the work of others and thinking of new possibilities. Although this research involved developing a vaccine, Jonas Salk considered himself an immunologist (a person who studies the immune system). As a researcher, he wanted to explore the immune system and the way it works. He believed this knowledge would help conquer viral diseases.

Independence Surfaces

In 1946 Salk was promoted to assistant professor in the department of epidemiology. Although Salk had

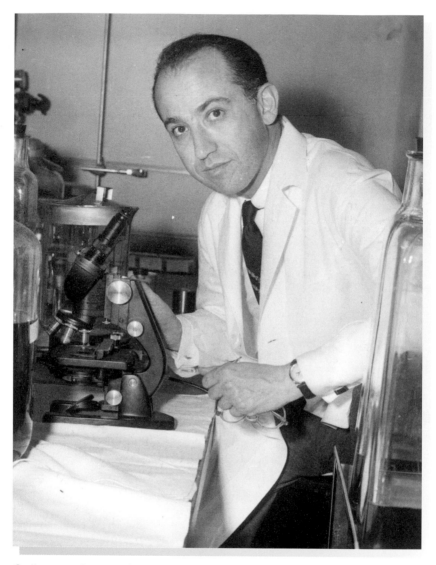

Salk examines animal tissue under a microscope.

been anxious to receive a university position, it came too late. He had grown restless and wanted more independence than his relationship with Francis allowed. In truth, Salk longed for his own laboratory and freedom to act on his own thinking. Salk later recalled, "I wanted to do independent work and I wanted

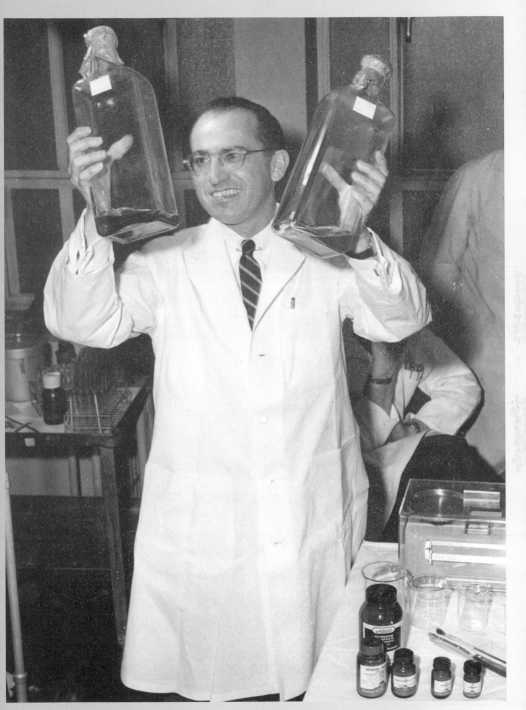

Salk holds up bottles used for growing poliovirus at the
University of Pittsburgh.

to do it *my way*."[6] With this in mind, he began looking for a position at a university where he could have his own laboratory.

Opportunity in Pittsburgh

About that time, Dr. William S. McEllroy, dean of the University of Pittsburgh School of Medicine, invited Salk to come to Pittsburgh. Although the school did not have a reputation as a leading research facility, Salk saw an opportunity to establish his own lab and develop his own research program. He later said, "I guess I fell in love . . . with . . . the prospect of independence."[7] Armed with this desire for independence and a strong will, Jonas Salk accepted the position and moved his family to Pittsburgh in October 1947.

Chapter Three

Conquering Hero

A t the University of Pittsburgh, Salk expected to find himself at the head of his own lab with the freedom to set up an independent research program. Instead, he was employed by the physics department under the supervision of Dr. Max A. Lauffer. To make matters worse, Lauffer worked with viruses that attacked plants while Salk's research involved viruses that attacked animals. Salk said later that "these two interests did not necessarily coincide [go together], to put it mildly."[8]

Salk thought he would have a large facility occupying empty floors he had seen in Pittsburgh's Municipal Hospital, across the street from the university. The area assigned to Salk for his lab, however, turned out to be a forty-by-forty-foot section in the basement that had once been the hospital's morgue. And the limited funds offered by the university would not equip the lab for the research Salk wanted to do.

NFIP had also noticed the unused space in Pittsburgh's Municipal Hospital. In fact, that empty space

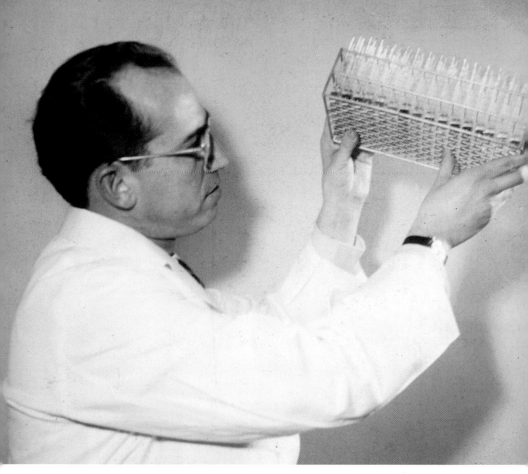

Salk inspects vials of serum used in polio research.

and NFIP's knowledge of Salk's work in influenza research at the University of Michigan would provide Salk with his dream laboratory and bring him into polio research.

Opportunity Knocks

By 1946 researchers had identified three types of **poliovirus**. No one knew if these were the only types of poliovirus that caused the disease. And no one knew how many poliovirus types a vaccine would have to contain to offer protection against all three types of polio. NFIP decided to find out. They set out to find four laboratories with four directors to conduct a poliovirus-typing program. In addition, they wanted to draw Dr. Jonas Salk into poliovirus research. They hoped the offer of thousands of dollars in laboratory funding for this program would do the job. It did.

Salk accepted NFIP's offer in 1948. He later explained that "it was an opportunity to learn something about polio, get facilities that I could do other things with, and assemble an adequate staff."[9] In addition, the virus-typing work might lead to the development of a vaccine.

With a $200,000 research grant from NFIP for laboratory equipment and operation, Salk was able to attract additional funding for remodeling the hospital floors. Between 1949 and 1955, Salk expanded his virus research

Salk (center) accepted a $200,000 research grant from members of the National Foundation for Infantile Paralysis.

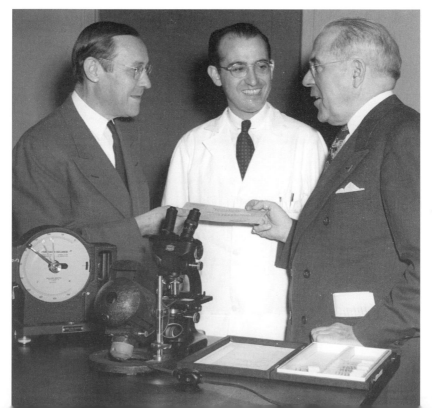

laboratory. The lab took up three floors of Municipal Hospital and employed more than fifty people.

Monkey Research

Poliovirus typing involved infecting a laboratory monkey with a known type of the virus, for example, Type I.

After the monkey became ill, it's body created antibodies to attack Type I poliovirus. When the monkey recovered, it would be immune to the disease caused by Type I poliovirus. That immune monkey would then be infected with an unknown type of poliovirus. If the monkey remained well, this identified the unknown poliovirus as Type I. If the monkey became ill with polio, the unknown poliovirus was then used to infect a monkey that had recovered from Type II virus. If the monkey remained well, the virus was identified as Type II; if it became ill, the virus was identified as Type III.

The virus typing was time-consuming and boring. It involved watching monkeys become ill, watching them recover, and watching them become ill again. Progress was slow. Each experiment took several weeks. Researchers waited for the virus to grow. They waited for the results of the experiments. And they waited to compare the results from one lab with the results from another lab. As time passed, Salk grew impatient to find a faster and better way.

Virus-Typing Shortcut

In 1949 another researcher, Dr. John F. Enders, discovered that poliovirus could be grown in laboratory

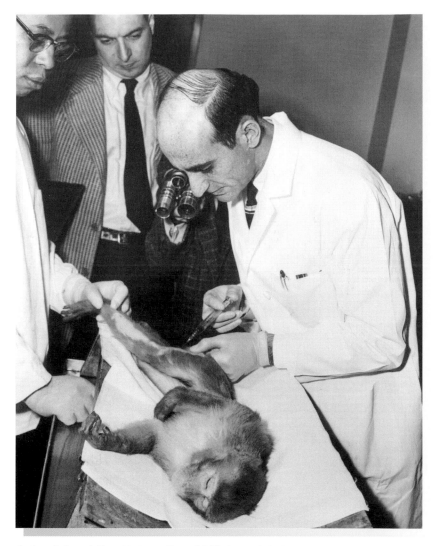

Scientists at the University of Pittsburgh inject a monkey with the polio vaccine.

test tubes in **culture medium** used to grow chickenpox virus. Other researchers paid little attention. Salk, however, immediately saw the possibilities of Enders's discovery. And, although others thought it could not be done, Salk envisioned a shortcut to virus typing. In his own research, he grew the virus in test tubes containing growing cells and culture medium. In the test tubes, he could then carry out virus-typing experiments with antibodies. Instead of waiting weeks for monkeys to become paralyzed he only had to wait days to see if the cells lived or died. For example, if Type I antibodies attacked the virus, this meant the unknown poliovirus was Type I.

Ready to Begin

By the fall of 1949, results from all four labs showed that no poliovirus had been found that did not fit into one of the three known types. Supporting these results with his own test-tube research data, Salk had seen enough evidence. He was convinced that a polio vaccine would have to contain only three strains of virus, one for each type. In addition, Enders's discovery made it possible to grow large amounts of poliovirus rapidly. This poliovirus could be killed and safely used

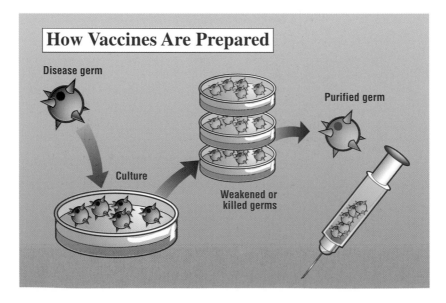

How Vaccines Are Prepared

Disease germ

Culture

Weakened or killed germs

Purified germ

for a vaccine. All Salk needed now was a way to kill *all* the virus in a batch and yet leave it in a form the body's immune system would recognize. Salk believed this would trigger the production of antibodies. He experimented with different formulas for killing the virus. He said, "When you try 30 variables [combinations], you're sure to hit the right one."[10] He then did extensive testing of every batch to be sure all the virus had been killed. When he found a way to kill *all* the virus in a batch, he was ready to begin work on a vaccine.

Development of the Vaccine

Salk received grants for his polio vaccine research from NFIP in July 1950. He began actual work on the killed virus vaccine in 1951. He tested the first batches of vaccine on monkeys. In the spring of 1952, he was so sure the vaccine was safe and effective that he injected it into his wife and three young sons.

Salk had a vaccine ready for clinical trials—that is, widespread human testing—in April 1954. NFIP tested the vaccine that summer. Of the 1,830,000 children who took part in the test, 440,000 received the vaccine, 210,000 received a dummy vaccination, and 1,180,000 unvaccinated children were observed. Very few of the children who received the vaccine came down with polio. When the results of the test were announced April 12, 1955, the public was told that the vaccine was up to 90 percent effective in preventing polio. After a brief weekend of celebration and interviews, Salk told reporters that "the most important thing to me is to get back in the

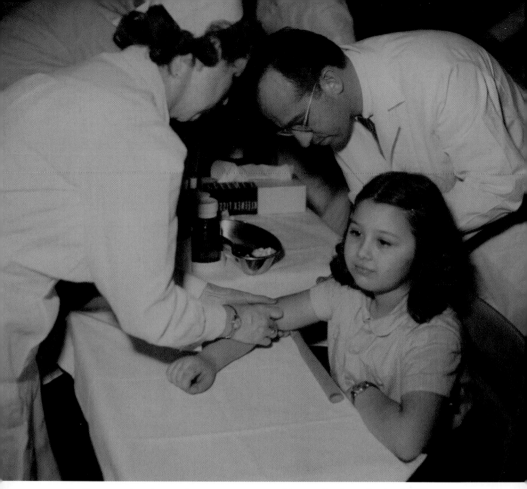

Salk vaccinates a brave young girl against polio in 1955.

lab."[11] Ninety percent was not good enough for Salk; he wanted to make the vaccine 100 percent effective. And he told the world he believed it could be done.

To Salk's peers, fellow doctors and scientists, this sounded like boasting. They thought he was taking credit for an achievement he should have been sharing with others, such as Enders and Salk's research team. In the hearts of most Americans, however, Jonas Salk was, and still is, the conquering hero who saved the children from polio.

Chapter Four

The Salk Legacy

Salk received some criticism from other scientists for doing research his own way. Interested in developing a vaccine to stop polio epidemics, he did not take time to publish the results of his research in medical journals before moving ahead. In the view of some other scientists, this meant Salk had taken shortcuts in his research. In Salk's view, however, he had used creative thinking to develop a better and faster, yet accurate, way to develop a safe vaccine.

No Patent

Salk's vaccine brought widespread recognition and public gratitude; however, it brought him no additional income. Neither Salk nor NFIP sought a patent and the formula was offered free to any pharmaceutical company equipped to produce it. After the success of the vaccine testing was announced, noted broadcaster Edward R. Murrow asked Salk who owned the patent on his vaccine. Salk answered that the vaccine belonged to the people and then added, "There is no

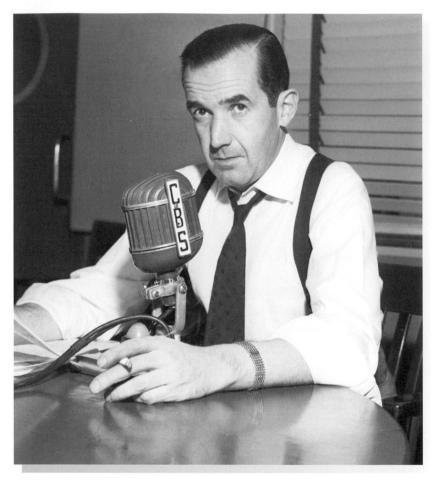

Broadcaster Edward R. Murrow interviewed Salk shortly after successful testing of the polio vaccine was completed.

patent. Could you patent the sun?"[12] The *Toronto Daily Star*, a Canadian newspaper, called the vaccine a gift to the world. And, as far as Jonas Salk and his staff were concerned, it was.

Awards

Salk had a creative mind. He was independent and did research in his own way. This displeased other scientists. As a result, they withheld some scientific awards from him. Still, Salk received many awards for his achievement, including a citation from President Dwight D. Eisenhower and the Congressional Medal of Honor for Distinguished Civilian Service. Many scholarship programs were created in his honor and universities gave him honorary degrees. He continued to receive recognition for his work after his death. In May 1999, the U.S. Postal Service issued a first-class postage stamp honoring Salk. In choosing the recipient of this honor, the Postal Service asked the American people what they considered to be the most

Salk proudly displays a presidential citation honoring his work on the polio vaccine.

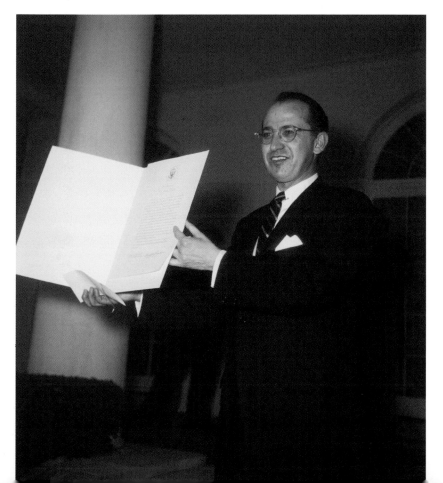

important science and technology advancement of the 1950s. They overwhelmingly answered the polio vaccine.

Dedicated to Research Until the End

Most people would consider the development of the first successful polio vaccine an accomplishment of a lifetime. Salk's success, however, came at the age of forty. Still a young man, he continued his poliovirus research, seeking an improved polio vaccine. He wanted to make the vaccine 100 percent effective.

When the threat of polio seemed over, he continued his work in immunology. He directed his life-long research toward finding cures and preventions for cancer, multiple sclerosis, and other diseases of the immune system. Success eluded him in his battles against these diseases. He founded the Salk Institute for Biological Studies in San Diego, California, to continue this research. In the mid-1980s, after the age of 70, he joined the battle against AIDS. He continued his work on a limited basis until his death from heart failure on June 23, 1995. He died in La Jolla, California, where he made his home with his second wife, Francoise, in his later years.

Salk's Legacy

Jonas Salk's gift to the world began with the polio vaccine. He opened the way for other scientists to bring their dreams to reality, to dare to think about possibilities, and pursue them. He truly believed that scientific

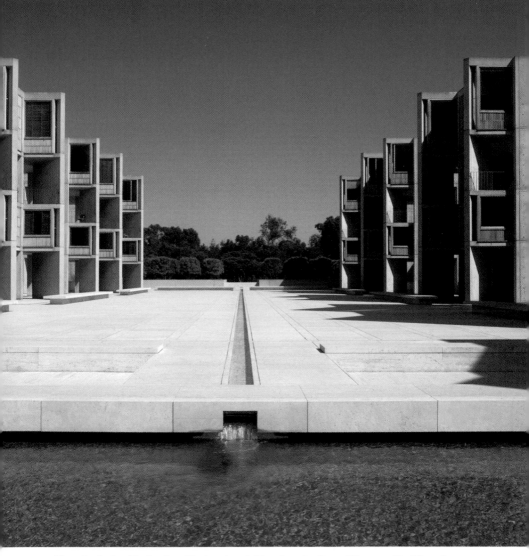

The Salk Institute for Biological Studies in San Diego, California, is dedicated to ongoing scientific discovery.

discoveries came from creative thinking. And he believed that a researcher must be free to work in his own way and follow his own instincts.

In 1963, Jonas Salk's dream of a laboratory where scientists could do things their own way became a reality. Today, the Salk Institute for Biological Studies stands as a monument to Salk's creativity. Its two beautifully designed buildings face each other on the cliffs at Torrey Pines, north of San Diego, California. Salk thought of the institute as a place to bring science and creativity together. He said, "I thought how nice it would be if a place like this existed and I was invited to work there."[13]

With grants from organizations such as NFIP and others, he built his dream laboratory and invited other researchers to follow their dreams, too. Salk believed that scientific discoveries were once someone's dream.

Salk stands on a rocky cliff overlooking the Pacific Ocean near his home in La Jolla, California.

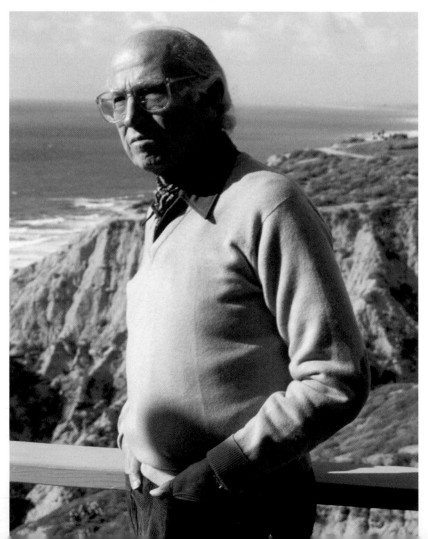

In his view, a cure for cancer, multiple sclerosis, or AIDS may be a young researcher's dream today. Someday soon that dream may be a reality. And the cure may be found at the Salk Institute.

Had Jonas Salk gone into private practice he could have been wealthy. He would have treated the sick and possibly saved hundreds of lives. As a research scientist, however, he helped conquer polio. In doing so, he kept millions of children from being crippled for life and prevented an untold number of deaths. Salk also set an example for other scientists to follow—to dream of possibilities and use creative thinking to make those possibilities real.

Notes

Chapter 1: A Boy with Potential

1. Quoted in Richard Carter, *Breakthrough: The Saga of Jonas Salk*. New York: Trident Press, 1966, p. 3.
2. Quoted in George Johnson, "Once Again a Man with a Mission," *New York Times Magazine*, November 25, 1990, p. 57.
3. Quoted in "Closing In on Polio," *Time,* March 29, 1954, p. 60.

Chapter 2: Man of Opportunity

4. Quoted in Carter, *Breakthrough*, p. 36
5. Quoted in Carter, *Breakthrough*, p. 48
6. Quoted in Carter, *Breakthrough*, p. 51
7. Quoted in Carter, *Breakthrough*, p. 53

Chapter 3: Conquering Hero

8. Quoted in Carter, *Breakthrough*, p. 55
9. Quoted in Carter, *Breakthrough*, p. 62
10. Quoted in "Closing In on Polio," p. 65.
11. Quoted in "It Works," *Time*, April 25, 1955, p. 52.

Chapter 4: The Salk Legacy

12. Quoted in Carter, *Breakthrough*, p. 284.
13. Quoted in Johnson, "Once Again a Man with a Mission," p. 61.

Glossary

antibodies: Proteins produced by the body's immune system that attack invading bacteria and viruses. The immune system custom designs antibodies to fight each invader it detects.

culture medium: A carefully balanced mixture designed to nourish the growth of bacteria and viruses in laboratories.

immune: A person is immune to a disease when his or her body has produced antibodies that destroy the bacteria or virus that causes that disease. They are protected from becoming ill from that disease.

infantile paralysis: Polio. A disease caused by a virus that in its worst form attacks the central nervous system and paralyzes the victim. Most of the victims are children.

killed virus vaccine: A vaccine that is made from virus that have been killed in such a way that the body recognizes it as a threat and produces antibodies to fight it.

laboratory: The workplace of a scientist that is designed and equipped to carry out research experiments.

live virus vaccine: A vaccine that is made from live virus that are too weak to cause the disease but will trigger the production of antibodies to protect against a disease.

poliovirus: Several strains of virus that cause polio-myelitis, sometimes known as infantile paralysis or polio.

vaccine: A fluid that is introduced into the body, usually with a needle, that causes the body to produce antibodies that protect the person from a disease.

For Further Exploration

Books

Jim Hargrove, *The Story of Jonas Salk and the Discovery of the Polio Vaccine.* Chicago: Childrens Press, 1990. A biography of Jonas Salk focusing on the discovery of the vaccine.

Peg Kehret and Denise Shanahan, *Small Steps: The Year I Got Polio.* Morton Grove, IL: Albert Whitman, 2000. The author recalls her battle against polio when she was thirteen and her struggle to overcome its effects.

Lydia Weaver and Aileen Arrington, *Close to Home: A Story of the Polio Epidemic.* New York: Penguin USA, 1997. A story about a young girl whose summer fun is overshadowed by a spreading polio epidemic in 1952 while her mother works with other scientists to develop a polio vaccine.

Periodicals

Renee Skelton, "Conquering Polio," *National Geographic World*, May 2000. A magazine article offering an overview of polio and the battle to conquer it.

Websites

Polio: Death of a Disease. www.philly.com/packages/polio. This site covers polio after the disease was controlled. It includes stories of people who had polio—some were poster children for the March of Dimes—

plus general information with links to video clips and a timeline.

A Brief History of Polio. http://128.59.173.136/PICO/Chapters/History.html. A detailed history of polio that includes a photo of a National Foundation of Infantile Paralysis brochure recommending dos and don'ts to follow during polio season.

A Short Timeline of Polio History. www.pbs.org/storyofpolio/polio/timeline/index.html. This site includes clickable thumbnails in a timeline beginning with the first epidemic in the United States in 1916. Clicking on the thumbnails brings up a larger photo with text giving details of the event.

Epidemic! On the Trail of Killer Diseases—Polio: A Terror About to Be Conquered. www.discovery.com/exp/epidemic/polio/polio.html. An overview of polio epidemics and the search for a vaccine. Includes coverage of Salk's development of the vaccine.

Index

Picture Credits

About the Author

Deanne Durrett has been writing nonfiction books for kids since 1993. She writes on a variety of subjects but her favorites are biographies. She loves research. To her it is an adventure filled with discovery. She and her husband Dan live in Arizona with Einstein (a mini schnauzer) and Willie (an Abyssinian cat). In her spare time, Ms. Durrett chooses from a variety of activities including playing computer games, and watching the rabbits and quail outside her window.